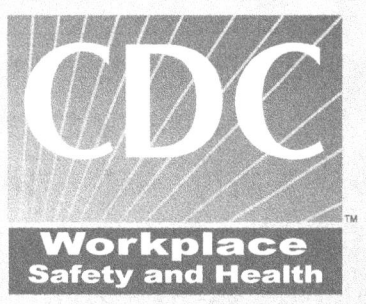

Metalworking Fluid Exposure at an Aircraft Engine Manufacturing Facility – Ohio

Lilia Chen, MS, CIH
Francisco Meza, MD, MPH
Naomi Hudson, Dr PH, MPH

Health Hazard Evaluation Report
HETA 2010-0144-3164
August 2012

DEPARTMENT OF HEALTH AND HUMAN SERVICES
Centers for Disease Control and Prevention

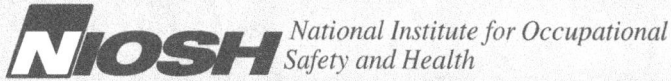

National Institute for Occupational
Safety and Health

The employer shall post a copy of this report for a period of 30 calendar days at or near the workplace(s) of affected employees. The employer shall take steps to insure that the posted determinations are not altered, defaced, or covered by other material during such period. [37 FR 23640, November 7, 1972, as amended at 45 FR 2653, January 14, 1980].

CONTENTS

ABBREVIATIONS

°C	Degrees Celsius
µm	Micrometer
ACGIH®	American Conference of Governmental Industrial Hygienists
BCYE	Buffered charcoal yeast extract
CFR	Code of Federal Regulations
CFU/mL	Colony forming units per milliliter
CI	Confidence interval
EU/m^3	Endotoxin unit per cubic meter
HHE	Health hazard evaluation
HP	Hypersensitivity pneumonitis
LEV	Local exhaust ventilation
Lpm	Liters per minute
MDC	Minimum detectable concentration
mg/m^3	Milligrams per cubic meter
mm	Millimeter
MQC	Minimum quantifiable concentration
MWF	Metalworking fluid
NAICS	North American Industry Classification System
NIOSH	National Institute for Occupational Safety and Health
OEL	Occupational exposure limit
OSHA	Occupational Safety and Health Administration
PBZ	Personal breathing zone
PPE	Personal protective equipment
PEL	Permissible exposure limit
PR	Prevalence ratio
REL	Recommended exposure limit
TLV®	Threshold limit value
TWA	Time-weighted average
VTL	Vertical turret lathe
WEEL™	Workplace environmental exposure level

HIGHLIGHTS OF THE NIOSH HEALTH HAZARD EVALUATION

The National Institute for Occupational Safety and Health (NIOSH) received a request from the United Automobile, Aerospace & Agricultural Implement Workers of America to evaluate exposure to metalworking fluids (MWFs) at an aircraft engine manufacturing facility in Ohio. The requestors were concerned about possible health hazards from a new MWF formulation.

What NIOSH Did

- We visited the facility in September 2010 and again in May 2011.

- We asked employees who did and did not work with MWFs to fill out a questionnaire about their medical and work history.

- We took air samples for MWFs and endotoxin and bulk samples of MWF for microbials.

- We reviewed the MWF maintenance and training programs.

- We assessed engineering controls (including ventilation). We also looked at work practices.

What NIOSH Found

- Employees who worked with MWFs reported more work-related asthma symptoms and dermatitis than employees who did not work with MWFs.

- All airborne MWF concentrations were very low. These levels were below applicable occupational exposure limits.

- Concentrations of endotoxin in the air were very low. These levels were below recommended guidelines.

- The central MWF supply systems had good microbial control.

- Some employees did not use splash guards, enclosures, and mist collectors when machines were in use.

- The preventive maintenance schedule for the mist collectors was not always followed.

What Managers Can Do

- Start a medical surveillance program for employees who are exposed to MWFs.

- Ensure that employees use engineering controls appropriately. These engineering controls can help control employees' exposure to MWFs.

- Follow a preventive maintenance schedule for the mist collectors.

- Have employees who work with MWFs wear protective sleeves.

- Train employees on MWF health hazards, use of personal protective equipment, and proper hygiene.
- Remind employees to report health concerns to their manager.
- Refer employees with possible work-related respiratory or skin problems to a physician. The physician should be knowledgeable about occupational exposures such as MWFs.

What Employees Can Do

- Leave mist collectors on and completely close machine enclosures.
- Use splash guards to contain splashing and misting.
- Tell your manager about any injuries or health concerns related to your work.
- Take any training that applies to your job when it is offered.
- Use personal protective equipment, such as gloves and protective sleeves, to keep MWFs off your skin.
- Wash MWFs off your skin with soap and water as soon as possible.
- Maintain good skin health through proper hygiene and use of moisturizers.

SUMMARY

MWF-exposed participants reported significantly higher rates of work-related asthma symptoms and work-related dermatitis symptoms in the last 12 months than participants not exposed to MWF. MWF and endotoxin concentrations were very low and below applicable occupational exposure limits. Low bacteria counts in the bulk MWF samples collected from the central MWF supply systems indicated good microbial control. A medical surveillance program and a healthy skin program are recommended for early identification and prevention of health symptoms.

In July 2010, NIOSH received a request for an HHE from a representative of the United Automobile, Aerospace & Agricultural Implement Workers of America to evaluate exposure to MWFs in an aircraft engine manufacturing facility in Ohio. The evaluation focused on workers exposed to a new formulation of a semisynthetic MWF introduced in January 2010.

We administered questionnaires to employees who worked with MWFs and to employees who did not use MWFs. The questionnaire asked about demographics, workplace practices and location, cigarette smoking, and skin and respiratory symptoms. We performed area and PBZ air sampling for MWF aerosols (thoracic particulate mass and extracted MWF) in the areas fed by the three central MWF supply systems. We also performed area air sampling for endotoxin. Bulk samples from the central MWF supply systems were collected for microbial analysis. We looked at the results of MWF tests done regularly at the facility. We also reviewed the company's MWF management program, PPE program, training materials, and material safety data sheets.

We found that MWF-exposed participants reported significantly higher rates of work-related asthma symptoms and of work-related dermatitis symptoms in the last 12 months than participants not exposed to MWFs. All airborne MWF concentrations were below applicable occupational exposure limits. Airborne endotoxin concentrations were below recommended guidelines. Low bacteria counts in bulk samples from the central MWF supply systems indicated good microbial control.

We recommended training employees on how to properly use engineering controls, such as mist collectors, machine partitions, enclosures, and splash guards. Management should ensure that the mist collector preventive maintenance scheduled is followed. The MWF management program should include better documentation of processes and procedures. This program should include information on employee training, environmental monitoring, and medical screening. A medical surveillance program should be started. It should include pre-employment and periodic questionnaires about respiratory and dermal symptoms. Employees with symptoms should be evaluated by a medical professional who is trained in occupational health. A healthy skin program should be started, which should include teaching employees about proper cleansing and use of protective sleeves.

Keywords: NAICS 336412 (Aircraft Engine and Engine Parts Manufacturing), metalworking fluid, MWF, thoracic particulates, asthma, dermatitis, endotoxin, mycobacteria, microbial contamination, fungi, aircraft engine manufacturing

NIOSH received a request for an HHE from the United Automobile, Aerospace & Agricultural Implement Workers of America to evaluate the possible health hazards of exposure to MWFs used as a coolant at an aircraft engine manufacturing facility in Ohio. In January 2010, a new formulation of a semisynthetic MWF was introduced. This product had lower foaming properties than the previous formulation. The new MWF was used in the three central MWF supply systems that fed approximately 275 machines in one large building.

Various types of aircraft engines were manufactured in a 70-year-old, one-story facility of approximately one million square feet. Approximately 360 employees worked in 11 cells (areas) over three shifts. Most machines in these cells were served by three central MWF supply systems: north, south, and shaft. These systems used approximately 20,000 gallons of MWFs. Machining operations included grinding, cutting, milling, and drilling. The most common machines on the production floor were VTLs, which remove material from a rotating work piece with cutting tools, mills, and drills. Other machines on the production floor included turning centers and grinders. MWFs were used to cool the cutting tools and machined parts and to remove metal shavings. Several machines not connected to the central supply systems operated on their own stand-alone MWF system. The MWFs in these stand-alone systems had different formulations from those in the central supply systems and MWFs were selected on the basis of requirements for specific tasks.

Metalworking Fluids

MWFs are complex mixtures used to cool, lubricate, and remove metal chips from tools and parts during machining of metal stock. MWFs often contain other substances including biocides, corrosion inhibitors, metal fines, tramp oils, and biological contaminants [NIOSH 1998; Burton et al. 2012]. Inhalation of MWF aerosols may irritate the throat, nose, and lung and has been associated with chronic bronchitis, asthma, HP, and worsening of pre-existing respiratory problems [Burton et al. 2012]. HP is a spectrum of granulomatous, interstitial lung diseases that occurs after repeated inhalation and sensitization to one or more of a wide variety of microbial agents (i.e., bacteria, fungi, amoebae), animal proteins, and low-molecular weight chemical antigens

[CDC 1996; Kreiss and Cox-Ganser 1997; Zacharisen et al. 1998]. NIOSH recommends limiting exposures to MWF aerosols to 0.4 mg/m³ for the thoracic particulate mass, as a TWA concentration for up to 10 hours per day during a 40-hour workweek [NIOSH 1998]. Detailed information on OELs is presented in Appendix A.

Skin contact with MWFs may cause allergic contact dermatitis or irritant contact dermatitis depending on the chemical composition, additives and contaminants, type of metal being machined, and the exposed individual's tendency for developing allergies [WISHA 2001].

Synthetic, semisynthetic, and soluble oil MWFs are diluted with water, so bacteria may grow if an inadequate amount of biocide is present. The Health and Safety Executive in the United Kingdom states that well-maintained MWFs have bacterial concentrations below 10^3 CFU/mL of fluid [HSE 2006]. Concentrations between 10^3 and 10^6 CFU/mL indicate reasonable control, and concentrations greater than 10^6 CFU/mL indicate poor control [HSE 2006]. The outer cell walls of Gram-negative bacteria may release lipopolysaccharide compounds called endotoxin when the bacteria die or multiply. Endotoxin is believed to cause adverse respiratory effects such as chronic bronchitis and asthma. In 2010, the Dutch Expert Committee on Occupational Safety recommended a health-based occupational exposure limit for airborne endotoxin of 90 EU/m³ [DECOS 2010]. Contaminated water in MWFs may also contain fungi. Some fungi may infect susceptible hosts, such as immune compromised persons, and some fungi may cause HP. At this time, health data are insufficient to recommend a specific limit for fungal contamination in MWFs.

ASSESSMENT

Sampling for MWF, Endotoxin, and Microbials

Full-shift area and PBZ air samples for MWF aerosols (thoracic particulate mass and extracted MWF) were collected over 2 days of sampling. During the sampling periods, we noted the type of engineering and ventilation controls used, location of each sample (north, south, or shaft central systems), cutting method (carbide, ceramic, or both) and activity performed (e.g., milling or grinding). Because each participant was already wearing multiple air sampling pumps, we collected area endotoxin air samples at the employees' work stations. Background concentrations of endotoxin were collected in a meeting room of a separate building. Additional details about MWF and endotoxin sampling and analysis are included in Appendix B.

We collected bulk samples of MWFs from each of the central supply systems, unused MWFs, and the water that was mixed with the concentrated MWFs. Eight bulk MWF samples were collected and analyzed by culture for bacteria, mycobacteria (which has been associated with HP), and fungi by a commercial laboratory. Details on the culture media, incubation temperature, and incubation times are contained in Appendix B.

We reviewed reports of the routine tests for MWF parameters, material safety data sheets, the MWF management program, MWF training materials, and PPE programs.

Exposure Groups

We recruited employees from the first and second shifts in the aircraft engine manufacturing building who usually worked with MWFs in their current jobs (exposed) and employees in an adjacent building who did not work directly with MWFs (unexposed). Employees in the unexposed group did assembly work, packing, and shipping.

Questionnaire

Participating employees filled out a questionnaire about demographics, work practices and location, cigarette smoking, and dermal and respiratory symptoms. Other questions addressed use of LEV controls, PPE use, and hand hygiene. Data were analyzed by age, sex, smoking status, hours worked per week, work area, and job title. We compared risk factors and symptoms between the exposed and unexposed participants. A P value equal to or less than 0.05 was considered significant. A 95% CI that does not include one was considered significant. Detailed methods are presented in Appendix B.

Air Sampling for MWFs

On May 5-6, 2011, we collected 48 PBZ air samples (Table C1 in Appendix C) and nine area air samples (Table C2 in Appendix C) for MWFs. Each sample was analyzed for thoracic particulates and the extractable fraction of MWFs. Thoracic particulates include all dust and other aerosols in the air (such as bioaerosols) in addition to the MWFs. The extractable fraction represents the portion of the sample that was MWFs.

Overall, concentrations of thoracic particulates and extracted MWFs were very low and did not exceed the NIOSH REL for thoracic particulates of 0.4 mg/m^3. Of the 48 PBZ air samples collected, two were excluded because of missing information on the datasheets and wide sampling pump precalibration and postcalibration differences. Eighteen of 43 PBZ air samples analyzed for thoracic particulates were quantifiable and 25 had concentrations between the MDC and MQC. None of the air samples had quantifiable concentrations of extracted MWFs, and only 4 of 43 PBZ air samples had extracted MWF concentrations between the MDC and MQC. Three air samples were taken on employees who did not work directly with MWF from the central systems (e.g., worked on a machine on a stand-alone system or in hot oil flush), but their work stations were surrounded by machines that were on the central systems. These concentrations were comparable to those found in the other air samples (Table C1).

Machines with various control techniques (e.g., types of enclosures, mist collectors) and cutting methods were spread throughout the work area. Older machines had splash guards and were partially enclosed, whereas newer machines were typically fully enclosed and computer operated. Because employees were usually assigned to one or two machines at a time during their shift, we identified similar exposure groups to evaluate any differences in exposures on the basis of control technique. These groups were classified by machine enclosure (fully enclosed, partially enclosed, no enclosure), ventilation controls (mist collector used or not), and cutting method (carbide or ceramic). Employees reported that ceramic cutting was performed at faster speeds and could cause more misting of MWFs. We observed that samples with quantifiable concentrations of thoracic particulates were collected mostly at grinders and at machines that did only ceramic cutting, although only one or two samples were taken in each of these groups. Because no meaningful air sample concentration differences were observed and because the number of samples in some groups was low, we did not further analyze the data by similar exposure groups.

Area air samples for MWFs were taken to supplement the PBZ air samples. One area sample was placed next to the north central system tank, two were obtained in areas where ceramic cutting was done by multiple machines close to each other, and one was taken in a different building (where the unexposed participants worked). The thoracic particulate air concentrations measured were similar to those in the PBZ air samples. No extracted MWF samples were quantifiable; two had concentrations between the MDC and MQC (Table C2).

Endotoxin

We took 20 area air samples for endotoxin throughout the plant. Two samples were taken in a meeting room in a completely separate area; one of these samples contained insufficient information so it is not reported (Table C3 in Appendix C). Endotoxin concentrations in the areas with MWF use ranged from 0.42 EU/m^3 to 2.7 EU/m^3 with a mean of 1.2 EU/m^3. The meeting room sample concentrations were 0.23 EU/m^3 and 0.24 EU/m^3. Because all concentrations were very low and did not vary widely, we did not analyze results further by similar exposure groups.

Microbials

Two bulk samples from each of the central systems were collected for microbial analysis. An unused sample of MWFs mixed from concentrated MWFs and deionized water to the manufacturer's recommended concentration, and a sample of the deionized water used to dilute the MWFs were also collected and analyzed (Table 1). The highest bacteria counts were in the south central system and ranged from 3 to 401 CFU/mL. Two types of bacteria were found in the deionized water. Our results showed that all bacterial concentrations were low, below 103 CFU/mL of fluid. The deionized water also contained four types of fungi. Although the shaft central system had no bacteria isolated, *Penicillium* spp. (a fungus) was isolated. The north and shaft central systems also had mycobacteria present. These mycobacteria were identified as a Ziehl-Neelsen stain species; however, the laboratory was unable to identify the exact species.

Table 1. Results from microbial analyses of bulk metalworking fluid samples

	Bacteria Isolated		Fungus Isolated		Mycobacteria
Location	Bacteria	(CFU/mL)	Fungus	(CFU/mL)	Presence
South branch	*Bacillus* spp.	100	None		None
	GNR, NF, morph* A	300			
	GNR, NF, morph* B	1			
South tank	GNR, NF, morph* B	10	*Penicillium* spp.	1	None
	GNR, NF, morph* C	10			
	GNR, NF, morph* D	100			
North tank	GNR, NF, morph* E	3	None		Present
North branch	None		None		Present
Shaft tank	None		*Penicillium* spp.	200	Present
Shaft branch	None		*Penicillium* spp.	2	Present
Deionized Water	*Corynebacterium* spp.	180	*Acremonium* spp.	3	None
	Aerobic actinomycetes	6	*Penicillium* spp.	2	
			Cladosporium spp.	100	
			Sterile hyaline mold	2	
Unused fluid (10.7% MWF)	None		None		None

*GNR, NF, morph = Gram-negative rod, non fermenter, morphotype

Bulk samples collected by the company at the same time as the NIOSH samples had similar results. However, the company's results showed higher bacteria counts (up to 4,000 CFU/mL). Fungi were not detected except in the deionized water sample (30 CFU/mL). Both sets of results showed that the deionized water used to dilute the MWF concentrate for the central systems had low levels of bacteria.

Other Observations

Overall, the production floor appeared to be clean, and visible mist was not present. The MWF maintenance program appeared to be comprehensive, but was not well documented, such as having a written standard operating procedure for testing the fluid. The coolant team met biweekly or as necessary, handled issues that arose concerning maintenance of the three central MWF supply systems, and oversaw activities of the contractor who performed daily maintenance of these systems. MWFs in the central systems were tested weekly for concentration, pH, conductivity, bacterial counts, percent free oil, fungal counts, total anaerobes, and amount of stabilizer. Our review of these results indicated that most of the parameters fell within the MWF manufacturer's recommended ranges. Parameters outside recommended ranges were bolded on the logs, and we were told that the MWF system contractor took necessary actions to rectify them in a timely manner.

Preventive maintenance activities, including filter changes on the mist collectors, were scheduled annually; however, we were told that due to resource limitations, some of these activities had not been completed as scheduled. We observed that some machines had mist collector systems, enclosures, and splash guards that operators did not always use when the machines were in use. In specific instances, enclosures and splash guards were not closed completely when the machines were in use. In other cases, mist collectors were not turned on.

PPE

Everyone in the manufacturing work area was required to wear safety glasses. However, we observed some employees not wearing safety glasses. This facility had a mandatory hearing conservation program for employees at machines where noise sampling performed by the company showed levels above the OSHA action level. Other employees used hearing protection voluntarily and only when needed. Earmuffs and a variety of ear plugs were available and stationed in various places in the work area. We observed that some ear plugs were not inserted fully in some employees' ears.

Employees were provided with a wide variety of gloves and barrier creams for dermal protection. These items were kept in a central location accessible to employees. We observed employees wearing nitrile, leather, or cut-resistant wrist-length gloves. We observed two employees not wearing gloves. We were told that for a few jobs that required fine manual manipulation, employees chose not to wear gloves because the gloves interfered with their work. Most employees wore short sleeve shirts. Uniforms were not required.

Questionnaire Results

Four hundred and seven employees completed the questionnaire. The participation rate was 82% (183/223) among the exposed group and 87% (224/257) among the unexposed group. Ninety-four percent of participants were aged 45 years or older (Table 2). The majority of both exposed and unexposed participants worked 41 hours or more per week. The proportion of participants who currently smoked was similar between groups, although more exposed participants were former smokers. The proportion of participants who were atopic (history of allergic symptoms such as allergic rhinitis, asthma, or eczema) was similar between exposed and unexposed.

Table 2. Demographic characteristics of participants by exposure group (n=407)

Characteristics	Total Number (%)	Exposed Number (%) n=183	Unexposed Number (%) n=224
Age			
18–24	2 (<1)	1 (1)	1 (<1)
25–34	11 (3)	—	11 (5)
35–44	10 (2)	5 (3)	5 (2)
45–54	163 (40)	88 (48)	75 (33)
55–64	212 (52)	83 (45)	129 (58)
65+	8 (2)	5 (3)	3 (1)
Unknown	1 (<1)	1 (1)	—
Sex			
Male	340 (84)	174 (95)	166 (74)
Female	67 (16)	9 (5)	58 (26)
Smoking Status			
Never	190 (47)	75 (41)	115 (51)
Former	152 (37)	79 (43)	73 (33)
Current	59 (15)	26 (14)	33 (15)
Unknown	6 (1)	3 (2)	3 (1)
Hours Worked/Week			
0–40 Hours	192 (47)	69 (36)	123 (55)
41+ Hours	214 (53)	113 (64)	101 (45)
Atopy	228 (56)	110 (60)	118 (53)

RESULTS
(CONTINUED)

The prevalence of dermatitis in the last 12 months was statistically significantly greater in the exposed group than in the unexposed group after controlling for atopy (Table 3). The most common location of dermatitis in both groups was the hands or fingers. Almost half of those reporting dermatitis in the past 12 months in both the exposed and unexposed groups reported having dermatitis currently. More exposed participants reported that their dermatitis symptoms were reduced with more than 5 days away from work (Table 3).

Table 3. Prevalence of dermatitis by MWF exposure category

	Exposed (n=183) Number (%)	Unexposed (n=224) Number (%)	PR (95% CI)
Dermatitis in the last 12 months	41 (22)	25 (11)	1.86 (1.20–2.90)
Location of dermatitis†			
Hands or fingers	30 (16)	21 (9)	1.61 (0.97–2.68)*
Wrists or forearm	20 (11)	9 (4)	2.45 (1.16–5.17)*
Face or neck	12 (7)	8 (4)	1.65 (0.70–3.90)*
Dermatitis currently	20 (11)	12 (5)	1.89 (0.96–3.72)
Dermatitis better when away from work more than 5 days	31 (17)	14 (6)	2.50 (1.39–4.49)
Changed job because of dermatitis	2 (1)	1 (<1)	2.15 (0.20–23.33)
Changed glove type or began wearing gloves because of dermatitis	15 (8)	0 (0)	—

*Adjusted for atopy
†Some participants reported more than one location of dermatitis

Exposed and unexposed participants were similar in frequency of glove use, but exposed participants were significantly more likely than unexposed to wear synthetic rubber (51% vs. 41%, $P = 0.049$) and leather gloves (49% vs. 27%, $P < 0.01$). Unexposed participants wore gloves to protect against cuts and abrasions during assembly work. Hand hygiene practices (use of barrier cream, hand washing, use of hand wipes or solvents to clean hands) did not differ significantly between exposed and unexposed participants. For the most part, hand hygiene practices, glove use, and glove type did not differ significantly between those who reported dermatitis on their hands or fingers or wrists or forearms in the last 12 months and those who did not (Table 4). However, participants with dermatitis on their hands or fingers or wrists or forearms in the last 12 months were significantly more likely to apply barrier cream at work (Table 4). Only 22% (9/41) of exposed participants with dermatitis in the last 12 months reported seeing a doctor for their dermatitis. Of these, none had patch testing.

Table 4. Hand hygiene practices and glove use by dermatitis on the hands or fingers, or wrists or forearms, in the last 12 months for exposed and unexposed participants combined

	Dermatitis in the last 12 months Number (%) n=58	No dermatitis in the last 12 months Number (%) n=348-349*	PR (95% CI)†
Applies barrier cream at work	12 (21)	20 (6)	4.64 (2.29-9.37)
Wash hands at least once per shift	58 (100)	345 (99)	—
Use hand-wipes to clean hands at least once per shift	33 (57)	186 (53)	1.13 (0.87–1.46)
Applies moisturizing lotion to hands or arms at work	31 (53)	190 (55)	0.98 (0.75–1.28)
Uses solvents to clean hands at work	8 (14)	24 (7)	2.23 (1.00–4.96)
Use gloves all of the time	19 (33)	90 (26)	1.33 (0.87–2.04)
Use gloves at least some of the time	56 (97)	320 (92)	1.07 (0.98–1.17)

*Denominators vary because of missing information
†Adjusted for atopy

RESULTS
(CONTINUED)

The proportion of participants who reported ever having asthma was similar between the exposed (11%) and unexposed groups (9%). About one third of those who reported ever having asthma reported that their asthma began during their current job. The prevalence of reported asthma symptoms by exposure group are in Table 5. These symptoms are taken from the European Community Respiratory Health Survey; a positive answer to any one indicates potential asthma (detailed information about the European Community Respiratory Health Survey can be found in Appendix B). The prevalence of work-related wheezing or whistling in the chest was significantly higher for the exposed than the unexposed participants (Table 5). The prevalence of participants who reported at least one asthma symptom and at least one work-related asthma symptom was significantly greater for participants exposed to MWFs than for unexposed participants after controlling for cigarette smoking status (Table 5). Because the REL is for a 40-hour work week, we compared the prevalence of asthma symptoms and work-related asthma symptoms between exposed participants who worked 40 hours per week or less and those who worked more than 40 hours per week. There was no significant difference between these groups.

The prevalence of sneezing, runny nose, or blocked nose was similar between exposed and unexposed participants; however, the prevalence of work-related nasal symptoms was significantly higher among the exposed (PR 1.36; CI: 1.003–1.86).

The prevalence of reported symptoms of HP by either of our definitions did not differ between exposed and unexposed participants. Six percent of exposed and unexposed participants reported one or more episodes of fever and weight loss in the last 12 months plus at least two of cough, wheeze, shortness of breath, or chest tightness. Less than 1% of participants in each group reported having pneumonia or chest flu more than twice in the last 12 months.

Table 5. Prevalence of asthma symptoms by exposure category*

Symptoms	Exposed (n=183) Number (%)	Unexposed (n=224) Number (%)	PR (95% CI)
Wheezing or whistling in chest†	46 (25)	35 (16)	1.54 (1.03–2.29)
Breathless when wheezing or whistling	18 (10)	19 (9)	1.13 (0.61–2.10)
Wheezing or whistling without a cold	37 (20)	26 (12)	1.66 (1.04–2.66)
Wheezing or whistling better on days off/vacation	32 (17)	14 (6)	2.84 (1.56–5.18)
Attack of asthma†	6 (3)	6 (3)	1.22 (0.40–3.76)
Attacks of asthma less often on days off/vacation	5 (3)	5 (2)	1.21 (0.35–4.13)
Woke up with feeling of tightness in chest†	26 (14)	13 (6)	2.47 (1.30–4.69)
Episodes of chest tightness less often on days off/vacation	18 (10)	10 (4)	2.22 (1.05–4.72)
Currently taking any medicine for asthma†	10 (5)	12 (5)	1.05 (0.46–2.39)
Take medicine less often on days off/vacation	5 (3)	3 (1)	2.28 (0.55–9.42)
Asthma symptoms‡	54 (30)	43 (19)	1.49 (1.05–2.13)
Work-related asthma symptoms	37 (20)	24 (11)	1.92 (1.19–3.09)

*Controlled for smoking status

†Derived from European Community Respiratory Health Survey; positive answer to any one indicates potential asthma

‡Asthma symptoms based upon a positive answer to one or more of four European Community Respiratory Health Survey questions

Discussion

Airborne MWF concentrations in this facility were generally well controlled, and none exceeded the NIOSH REL of 0.4 mg/m^3 for the thoracic particulate mass, as a TWA concentration for up to 10 hours per day during a 40-hour week. Because some employees reported working longer than 40 hours per week, this REL may be lowered by a reduction factor depending on the duration of exposure. We observed that samples with quantifiable concentrations of thoracic particulates were collected mostly at grinders and at machines that did only ceramic cutting. Although only one or two samples were taken in each of these similar exposure groups, other studies have found that grinding can generate higher concentrations of MWF mist than milling and turning [Simpson et al. 2003].

Mist collectors were installed on most of the machines that used MWFs. The mist collectors pulled air containing MWF mist from the area of the mist-generating activity through a high-efficiency particulate air filter and released the filtered air back into the work area. Mist collectors' performance degrades over time from various causes such as dust or contaminant buildup and mechanical failures. Therefore, if the filters are not replaced regularly and the performance parameters are not periodically checked, mist collectors lose the ability to maintain designed airflow requirements, which could expose workers to higher MWF concentrations. Adhering to a preventive maintenance plan to ensure optimum LEV performance will provide long-term worker protection from exposures and capitalize on the initial investment in the mist collectors [ACGIH 2007].

Wiring mist collectors so that they automatically turn on when the machine is in use would reduce the burden on the operator. Mist collectors should also be used as designed for optimum performance of drawing air contaminants away from the worker. If the machine's mist collector system was designed to be used with the enclosures in place, leaving the enclosures open could reduce capture efficiency and increase exposures.

The highest endotoxin concentration measured (2.7 EU/m^3) was well below the Dutch Expert Committee on Occupational Safety recommendation of 90 EU/m^3 for airborne endotoxin. Most of our endotoxin sampling results were much lower than those cited in other studies. Gilbert et al. found endotoxin levels ranging from 2.1 EU/m^3 to 183 EU/m^3 at 44 sites from 25 industries using MWFs in Quebec, Canada [Gilbert et al. 2010]. Another

DISCUSSION
(CONTINUED)

study measuring area endotoxin concentrations at a facility using semisynthetic MWFs in turning lathe and milling machining centers and a facility machining large and small parts using semisynthetic and synthetic MWFs found concentrations that ranged from 3.3 to 127 EU/m^3 [Wang 2007].

Our results showed good bacterial control in this facility based upon HSE recommendations of bacterial concentrations below 10^3 CFU/mL of fluid [HSE 2006]. The company's results showed good control overall because all bacterial counts fell below the 10^3 CFU/mL recommendation except for one sample. This sample had 4,000 CFU/mL, which indicated reasonable control [HSE 2006]. Mycobacteria of the Ziehl-Neelsen stain were present in the bulk samples, but the laboratory was unable to isolate the exact species for identification. Because mycobacteria have been found in MWFs in workplaces with HP outbreaks [Kreiss and Cox-Ganser 1997], bioaerosol control should be practiced to prevent the occurrence of HP [Passman et al. 2009].

Typically, fungi isolated from MWFs are common saprophytic species that live on decaying organic matter in the environment. Although present, fungi usually are not a major microbial contaminant in MWFs. The *Penicillium* species, which we found in the MWF in this facility, has been implicated in HP, but the relationship between fungal contamination and occupational asthma associated with MWF exposures is uncertain [NIOSH 1998].

While we did not find a difference in the occurrence of HP symptoms between exposed and unexposed employees, others have found cases of work-related HP in employees exposed to MWFs below the NIOSH REL [Kreiss and Cox-Ganser 1997]. The company's clinical staff was aware of HP in the past, but no cases had occurred recently. HP is rare and often misdiagnosed making it difficult to detect. Employees with fever, weight loss, cough, shortness of breath, wheeze, chest tightness, chest flu, or pneumonia should be evaluated by a healthcare provider knowledgeable about HP who can monitor symptoms to ensure early diagnosis and treatment.

Despite the low airborne concentrations of MWF, exposed participants were significantly more likely to report asthma symptoms and work-related asthma symptoms than unexposed participants. However, there was no significant difference when employees were asked if they ever had asthma. This might be due

Discussion
(continued)

to underdiagnosis of asthma; Milton et al. suggested that asthma is underreported in the workplace [Milton et al. 1998]. Case reports of occupational asthma have demonstrated that the NIOSH REL for MWFs did not consistently protect against allergic respiratory sensitization [Kreiss and Cox-Ganser 1997; Mapp et al. 2005]. NIOSH recognized that the REL might not be protective of all employees when it was developed [NIOSH 1998].

Contact dermatitis results from skin contact with MWFs and can be irritant, allergic, or both [Rom 2007]. Contact dermatitis is an inflammatory skin condition caused by skin contact with agents such as chemical irritants (irritant contact dermatitis) or allergens (allergic contact dermatitis). Irritant contact dermatitis is skin inflammation due to direct cell damage from a chemical or physical agent, while allergic contact dermatitis is a delayed immune reaction. Usually only a small percentage of people are susceptible to skin allergens. Exposed areas of skin, such as hands and forearms, have the greatest contact with irritants or allergens and are most commonly affected [Warshaw et al. 2003]. It is often impossible to clinically distinguish irritant contact from allergic contact dermatitis, as both can have a similar appearance and both can result in an acute, subacute, or chronic condition. Skin patch testing is required to distinguish between the two. In our evaluation, exposed participants were significantly more likely to report dermatitis in the last 12 months. Wrist and forearm dermatitis was significantly more prevalent among exposed participants, but hand dermatitis, while more common in exposed participants, was not significantly higher. We noted many employees wearing short sleeves, which may allow wrist and forearm contact with MWFs, while the hands are protected by gloves.

Frequency of glove use was similar between exposed and unexposed participants, and between those with and without dermatitis, but this does not rule out the possibility that glove use may be related to dermatitis for some employees in either group. Protective gloves can reduce or eliminate skin exposure to hazardous substances if used correctly, but may actually cause or worsen hand dermatitis (contamination by permeation and penetration) if selected poorly and used improperly [Foo et al. 2006]. Gloves may hold/keep irritants or allergens next to the skin [Kwon et al. 2006]. In addition, certain components of gloves are allergens themselves, and merely wearing gloves can lead to sweating and irritant dermatitis. Often if working in a water-tight glove, it is best to place a breathable cotton glove underneath

DISCUSSION (CONTINUED)

the occlusive glove. Similarly, the excessive pursuit of personal hygiene in the workplace may actually lead to misuse of soaps and detergents and cause irritant contact dermatitis. Proper hand washing methods and adequate moisturizing are valuable in preventing contact dermatitis [Warshaw 2003].

Those with dermatitis in our evaluation reported using barrier creams significantly more often than those without dermatitis. It is not clear if they were using the cream because they had dermatitis or if the dermatitis was caused or exacerbated by the barrier cream. The effectiveness of barrier creams is controversial. Evidence of the protective nature of these topical products during actual working conditions is limited [Schwantiz et al. 2003; Loffler et al. 2006; Weisshaar et al. 2006].

Solvents are able to dissolve grease and fat. When skin is exposed to solvents, solvents may remove the fat from the skin, causing dryness, scaling, and fissuring of the hands [Rom 2007]. Some solvents may also allow other chemicals to penetrate the skin more easily [OSHA 2008]. Solvents should not be used directly on the skin. Six percent of exposed participants and 5% of unexposed participants reported using solvents to clean their hands at work, but the prevalence of hand and finger dermatitis, and wrist and forearm dermatitis was higher among those exposed to MWFs.

Limitations of this work include the cross-sectional design of the evaluation. Cross-sectional studies collect information on exposures and health outcomes at the same time, so that causality cannot be proven. Industrial hygiene sampling can only document exposures on the days of sampling in the locations sampled. In addition, we did not perform clinical examinations to diagnose dermatitis and asthma. However, the European Community Respiratory Health Survey has a sensitivity of 75% and a specificity of 80% for asthma symptoms on the basis of a clinical examination with immunoglobulin E testing against common allergens, spirometry, and methacholine challenge testing [Grassi et al. 2003]. The dermatologic questions include standardized questions modified from the Nordic Occupational Skin Questionnaire [Susitaival et al. 2003], which is widely used in studies of dermatitis.

CONCLUSIONS

Participants exposed to MWFs reported significantly higher prevalence rates of work-related dermatitis and work-related asthma symptoms in the last 12 months than participants not exposed to MWFs. Dermal and respiratory symptoms were reported despite airborne exposure to MWFs below the REL. Following a preventive maintenance program for the mist collectors and appropriate use of engineering controls (i.e., machine enclosures, splash guards, mist collectors) will help lower airborne levels of MWFs. Instituting a medical surveillance program can provide earlier identification of potential problems.

RECOMMENDATIONS

On the basis of our findings, we recommend the actions listed below to create a more healthful workplace. We encourage you to use a labor-management health and safety committee or working group to discuss the recommendations in this report and develop an action plan. Those involved in the work can best set priorities and assess the feasibility of our recommendations for this specific situation. We also recommend referring to the OSHA document "Metalworking Fluids: Safety and Health Best Practices Manual" [OSHA 1999], which contains best practices to assist employers in providing safe and healthful workplace for workers exposed to MWF through effective prevention programs. Our recommendations are based on the hierarchy of controls approach (refer to Appendix A: Occupational Exposure Limits and Health Effects). This approach groups actions by their likely effectiveness in reducing or removing hazards. In most cases, the preferred approach is to eliminate hazardous materials or processes and install engineering controls to reduce exposure or shield employees. Until such controls are in place, or if they are not effective or feasible, administrative measures and/or PPE may be needed.

Engineering Controls

Engineering controls reduce exposures to employees by removing the hazard from the process or placing a barrier between the hazard and the employee. Engineering controls are very effective at protecting employees without placing primary responsibility of implementation on the employee.

1. Enforce the use of available engineering controls. Use partitions and splash guards as recommended by the machine manufacturer.

2. Wire mist collectors to automatically turn on when the machine is in use.

3. Prioritize and perform the scheduled preventive maintenance on the mist collectors. Refer to the *Industrial Ventilation Manual of Recommended Practice for Operation and Maintenance* for specific recommended practices for maintaining mist collector effectiveness [ACGIH 2007].

Administrative Controls

Administrative controls are management-dictated work practices and policies to reduce or prevent exposures to workplace hazards. The effectiveness of administrative changes in work practices for controlling workplace hazards is dependent on management commitment and employee acceptance. Regular monitoring and reinforcement are necessary to ensure that control policies and procedures are not circumvented in the name of convenience or production.

1. Improve documentation of the MWF management program. MWF management programs include a written standard operating procedure for testing MWF, a data collection and tracking system, safety and health training, exposure monitoring, employee participation, hazard prevention and control, and medical monitoring [OSHA 1999].

2. Maintain bacterial concentrations below 1,000 CFU/mL [HSE 2006]. Consider filtering bacteria from the deionized water used to mix with unused MWF.

3. Provide training on hand hygiene and ensure that employees do not wash hands with solvents.

4. Start a medical surveillance program for employees who are exposed to MWFs. At a minimum, use a medical questionnaire that focuses on skin and respiratory symptoms that may be work related. The questionnaire should be given prior to placement in a job with MWF exposure and periodically thereafter. In addition, employees should report work-related skin, eye, and respiratory symptoms to their supervisor. Employees who report work-related symptoms should be evaluated by a physician experienced in occupational medicine or allergy. If employees develop occupational rhinitis or asthma, they should be removed from exposure to MWF and placed in a job without MWF exposure while maintaining their earnings, seniority, and other rights and benefits.

5. Refer employees with recurrent or persistent skin symptoms in a timely manner to a dermatologist knowledgeable about occupational skin diseases and skin patch testing. Allergic contact dermatitis can be diagnosed definitively only with skin patch allergy testing. Skin patch testing allows these employees to know if they have skin allergy to certain workplace substances, as well as to other common skin allergens. The results can be used to counsel employees individually on what substances to avoid to prevent dermatitis recurrence. If these protective methods fail to relieve the dermatitis symptoms, then removal from exposure may be necessary. In some cases of allergic skin disease, employees may have to be reassigned to areas where exposure is minimal or nonexistent with retention of earnings, seniority, and other rights and benefits.

6. Provide annual healthy skin program training in the fall to help employees remember preventive measures they can take to protect their skin from drying out in winter. Employees with a history of allergic disease should be informed that they are at increased risk for developing contact dermatitis and need to take extra precautions to keep their skin healthy. See Appendix D for tips on preventing dermatitis. Healthy skin is one of the best protections against irritant and allergic contact dermatitis.

Personal Protective Equipment

PPE is the least effective means for controlling employee exposures. Proper use of PPE requires a comprehensive program and calls for a high level of employee involvement and commitment to be effective. The use of PPE requires the choice of the appropriate equipment to reduce the hazard and the development of supporting programs such as training, change-out schedules, and medical assessment if needed. PPE should not be relied upon as the sole method for limiting employee exposures. Rather, PPE should be used until engineering and administrative controls can be demonstrated to be effective in limiting exposures to acceptable levels.

1. Ensure gloves used by employees are appropriate for the task. Discontinue the use of natural rubber latex gloves. Natural rubber latex can lead to serious allergy (rhinitis, asthma, hives, and anaphylaxis).

RECOMMENDATIONS (CONTINUED)

2. Place a breathable cotton glove underneath non-breathable gloves.

3. Consider the use of protective sleeves to prevent MWFs from getting on wrists and forearms.

4. See Appendix D for tips on preventing dermatitis.

5. Provide additional training on the proper use of hearing protection.

REFERENCES

ACGIH [2007]. Industrial ventilation. A manual of recommended practice for operation and maintenance. Cincinnati, OH: American Conference of Governmental Industrial Hygienists.

Burton CM, Crook B, Scaife H, Evans GS, Barber CM [2012]. Systematic review of respiratory outbreaks associated with exposure to water based metalworking fluids. Ann Occup Hyg [epub online ahead of print - doi:10.1093/annhyg/mer121].

Centers for Disease Control and Prevention (CDC) [1996]. Biopsy-confirmed hypersensitivity pneumonitis in automobile production workers exposed to metalworking fluids - Michigan, 1994-1995. MMWR 45(28):606-610.

DECOS [2010]. Endotoxins: health-based recommended occupational exposure limit. The Hague: Health Council of the Netherlands, Dutch Expert Committee on Occupational Safety. [http://www.gezondheidsraad.nl/sites/default/files/201004OSH.pdf]. Date accessed: April 2012.

Foo CC, Goon AT, Leow YH, Goh CL [2006]. Adverse skin reactions to personal protective equipment against severe acute respiratory syndrome-a descriptive study in Singapore. Contact Dermatitis 55(5):291-294.

Gilbert Y, Veillette M, Meriaux A, Lavoie J, Cormier Y, Duchaine C [2010]. Metalworking fluid-related aerosols in machining plants. J Occup Environ Hyg 7(5):280-289.

Grassi M, Rezzani C, Biino G, Marinoni A [2003]. Asthma-like symptoms assessment through ECRHS screening questionnaire scoring. J Clin Epidemiol. 56(3):238-247.

References
(CONTINUED)

HSE (Health and Safety Executive) [2006]. Managing sumps and bacterial contamination - control approach 4. COSHH essentials for machining with metalworking fluids. [http://www.hse.gov.uk/pubns/guidance/mw05.pdf]. Date accessed: April 2012.

Kreiss K, Cox-Ganser J [1997]. Metalworking fluid-associated hypersensitivity pneumonitis: a workshop summary. Am J Ind Med 32(4):423–432.

Kwon S, Campbell LS, Zirwas MJ [2006]. Role of protective gloves in the causation and treatment of occupational irritant contact dermatitis. J Am Acad Dermatol 55(5):891–896.

Loffler H, Bruckner T, Diepgen T, Effendy I [2006]. Primary prevention in health care employees: a prospective intervention study with a 3-year training period. Contact Dermatitis 54(4):202–209.

Mapp CE, Boschetto P, Maestrelli P, Fabbri LM [2005]. Occupational asthma. Am J Respir Crit Care Med 172(3):280–305.

Milton DK, Solomon GM, Rosiello RA, Herrick RF [1998]. Risk and incidence of asthma attributable to occupational exposure among HMO members. Am J Ind Med 33(1):1–10.

NIOSH [1998]. Criteria for a recommended standard. Occupational exposure to metalworking fluids. Cincinnati, OH: U.S. Department of Health and Human Services, Centers for Disease Control and Prevention, National Institute for Occupational Safety and Health, Publication No. 98-102.

OSHA [1999]. Metalworking fluids: safety and health best practices manual. Washington, DC: U.S. Department of Labor, Occupational Safety and Health Administration. [http://www.osha.gov/SLTC/metalworkingfluids/metalworkingfluids_manual.html]. Date accessed: May 2012.

OSHA [2008]. OSHA technical manual. Washington, D.C.: Department of Labor, Occupational Safety and Health Administration, Section 2, Chapter 12. [http://www.osha.gov/dts/osta/otm/otm_ii/otm_ii_2.html]. Date accessed: April 2012.

Passman FJ, Rossmoore K, Roosmoore L [2009]. Relationship between the presence of mycobacteria and non-mycobacteria in metalworking fluids. Tribology & Lubrication Technology, pp. 52-55. [http://www.stle.org/assets/document/52_Mycobacteria.pdf]. Date accessed: April 2012.

Rom WN [2007]. Environmental and occupational medicine. 4th ed. Philadephia, PA: Lippincot Williams & Wilkins, pp. 620-627.

Schwanitz HJ, Riel U, Schlesinger T, Bock M, Skudlik C, Wulfhorst B [2003]. Skin care management: educational aspects. Int Arch Occup Environ Health 76(5):374-381.

Simpson AT, Stear M, Groves JA, Piney M, Bradley SD, Stagg S, Crook B [2003]. Occupational exposures to metalworking fluid mist and sump fluid contaminants. Ann Occup Hyg 47(1):17-30.

Susitaival P, Flyvholm MA, Meding B, Kanerva L, Lindberg M, Svensson A, Olafsson JH [2003]. Nordic Occupational Skin Questionnaire (NOSQ-2002): a new tool for surveying occupational skin diseases and exposure. Contact Dermatitis 49(2):70-76.

Wang H, Reponen T, Lee SA, White E, Grinshpun SA [2007]. Size distribution of airborne mist and endotoxin-containing particles in metalworking fluid environments. J Occup Environ Hyg 4(3):157-165.

Warshaw E, Lee G, Storrs FJ [2003]. Hand dermatitis: a review of clinical features, therapeutic options and long-term outcomes. Am J Contact Dermat 14(3):119-137.

Weisshaer E, Radulescu M, Bock M, Albrecht U, Diepgen TL [2006]. Educational and dermatological aspects of secondary individual prevention in healthcare workers. Contact Dermatitis 54(5):254-260.

WISHA [2001]. Preventing occupational dermatitis. Olympia, WA: Washington State Department of Labor and Industries, Safety & Health Assessment & Research for Prevention (SHARP) Publication No. 56-01-1999.

Zacharisen MC, Kadambi AR, Schlueter DP, Kurup VP, Shack JB, Fox JL, Anderson HA, Fink JN [1998]. The spectrum of respiratory disease associated with exposure to metal working fluids. J Occup Environ Med 40(7):640–647.

In evaluating the hazards posed by workplace exposures, NIOSH investigators use both mandatory (legally enforceable) and recommended OELs for chemical, physical, and biological agents as a guide for making recommendations. OELs have been developed by federal agencies and safety and health organizations to prevent the occurrence of adverse health effects from workplace exposures. Generally, OELs suggest levels of exposure that most employees may be exposed to for up to 10 hours per day, 40 hours per week, for a working lifetime, without experiencing adverse health effects. However, not all employees will be protected from adverse health effects even if their exposures are maintained below these levels. A small percentage may experience adverse health effects because of individual susceptibility, a preexisting medical condition, and/or hypersensitivity (allergy). In addition, some hazardous substances may act in combination with other workplace exposures, the general environment, or with medications or personal habits of the employee to produce adverse health effects even if the occupational exposures are controlled at the level set by the exposure limit. Also, some substances can be absorbed by direct contact with the skin and mucous membranes in addition to being inhaled, which contributes to the individual's overall exposure.

In the United States, OELs have been established by federal agencies, professional organizations, state and local governments, and other entities. Some OELs are legally enforceable limits, while others are recommendations. The U.S. Department of Labor OSHA PELs (29 CFR 1910 [general industry]; 29 CFR 1926 [construction industry]; and 29 CFR 1917 [maritime industry]) are legal limits enforceable in workplaces covered under the Occupational Safety and Health Act of 1970. NIOSH RELs are recommendations based on a critical review of the scientific and technical information available on a given hazard and the adequacy of methods to identify and control the hazard. NIOSH RELs can be found in the *NIOSH Pocket Guide to Chemical Hazards* [NIOSH 2010]. NIOSH also recommends different types of risk management practices (e.g , engineering controls, safe work practices, employee education/training, personal protective equipment, and exposure and medical monitoring) to minimize the risk of exposure and adverse health effects from these hazards. Other OELs that are commonly used and cited in the United States include the TLVs recommended by ACGIH, a professional organization, and the WEELs recommended by the American Industrial Hygiene Association, another professional organization. The TLVs and WEELs are developed by committee members of these associations from a review of the published, peer-reviewed literature. They are not consensus standards. ACGIH TLVs are considered voluntary exposure guidelines for use by industrial hygienists and others trained in this discipline "to assist in the control of health hazards" [ACGIH 2011]. WEELs have been established for some chemicals "when no other legal or authoritative limits exist" [AIHA 2011].

Outside the United States, OELs have been established by various agencies and organizations and include both legal and recommended limits. The Institut für Arbeitsschutz der Deutschen Gesetzlichen Unfallversicherung (IFA, Institute for Occupational Safety and Health of the German Social Accident Insurance) maintains a database of international OELs from European Union member states, Canada (Québec), Japan, Switzerland, and the United States. The database, available at http://www.dguv.de/ifa/en/gestis/limit_values/index.jsp, contains international limits for over 1,500 hazardous substances and is updated periodically.

Employers should understand that not all hazardous chemicals have specific OSHA PELs, and for some agents the legally enforceable and recommended limits may not reflect current health-based information. However, an employer is still required by OSHA to protect its employees from hazards even in the absence of a specific OSHA

PEL. OSHA requires an employer to furnish employees a place of employment free from recognized hazards that cause or are likely to cause death or serious physical harm [Occupational Safety and Health Act of 1970 (Public Law 91–596, sec. 5(a)(1))]. Thus, NIOSH investigators encourage employers to make use of other OELs when making risk assessments and risk management decisions to best protect the health of their employees. NIOSH investigators also encourage the use of the traditional hierarchy of controls approach to eliminate or minimize identified workplace hazards. This includes, in order of preference, the use of (1) substitution or elimination of the hazardous agent, (2) engineering controls (e.g., local exhaust ventilation, process enclosure, dilution ventilation), (3) administrative controls (e.g., limiting time of exposure, employee training, work practice changes, medical surveillance), and (4) personal protective equipment (e.g., respiratory protection, gloves, eye protection, hearing protection). Control banding, a qualitative risk assessment and risk management tool, is a complementary approach to protecting employee health that focuses resources on exposure controls by describing how a risk needs to be managed. Information on control banding is available at http://www.cdc.gov/niosh/topics/ctrlbanding. This approach can be applied in situations where OELs have not been established or can be used to supplement the OELs, when available.

Below we provide the OELs and surface contamination limits for the compounds we measured.

Metalworking Fluid

NIOSH recommends limiting exposures to MWF aerosols to 0.4 mg/m^3 for the thoracic particulate mass, as a TWA concentration for up to 10 hours per day during a 40-hour workweek [NIOSH 1998]. The NIOSH REL is intended to prevent or greatly reduce respiratory disorders associated with MWF exposure. Some employees have developed work-related asthma, HP, or other adverse respiratory effects when exposed to MWFs concentrations below the NIOSH REL. Limiting exposure to MWF aerosols is also prudent because certain MWF exposures have been associated with various cancers. In addition, limiting dermal (skin) exposure is critical to preventing allergic and irritant disorders related to MWF exposure. In most metalworking operations, it is technologically feasible to limit MWF aerosol exposures to 0.4 mg/m^3 or less. Medical monitoring is needed for the early identification of employees who develop symptoms of MWF-related conditions such as HP, asthma, and dermatitis.

Microbial Contaminants

Insufficient data exist to determine what constitutes a safe level of microbial contamination in MWF – either in terms of species present, absolute number of colony forming units, or microbial components, such as endotoxin. The Health and Safety Executive has suggested that well-maintained MWFs should have bacterial concentrations below 10^3 CFU/mL of fluid [HSE 2006]. Concentrations between 10^3 and 10^6 CFU/mL indicate reasonable control; control measures should be reviewed control and lower bacteria. Concentrations greater than 10^6 CFU/mL indicate poor control, and immediate action should take place, including draining and cleaning the system if necessary [HSE 2006]. At this time there is insufficient health data to recommend a specific limit for fungal contamination in MWF.

Rylander and Jacobs have suggested an occupational threshold concentration equivalent to 100 EU/m^3 of air to prevent airway inflammation [Rylander and Jacobs 1997]. No accepted occupational exposure limits have been developed in the United States because of the variability of sampling and analytical methods, and because of a lack of data showing a consistent dose-response relationship. In 2010, the Dutch Expert Committee on Occupational Safety recommended a health-based occupational exposure limit for airborne endotoxin of 90 EU/m^3 as an 8-hour TWA [DECOS 2010].

References

ACGIH [2011]. 2011 TLVs® and BEIs®: threshold limit values for chemical substances and physical agents and biological exposure indices. Cincinnati, OH: American Conference of Governmental Industrial Hygienists.

AIHA [2011]. AIHA 2011 emergency response planning guidelines (ERPG) & workplace environmental exposure levels (WEEL) handbook. Fairfax, VA: American Industrial Hygiene Association.

CFR. Code of Federal Regulations. Washington, DC: U.S. Government Printing Office, Office of the Federal Register.

DECOS [2010]. Endotoxins: health-based recommended occupational exposure limit. The Hague: Health Council of the Netherlands, Dutch Expert Committee on Occupational Safety. [http://www.gezondheidsraad.nl/sites/default/files/201004OSH.pdf]. Date accessed: April 2012.

HSE (Health and Safety Executive) [2006]. Bacterial contamination. [http://www.hse.gov.uk/metalworking/bacterial.htm]. Date accessed: April 2012.

NIOSH [1998]. Criteria for a recommended standard: Occupational exposure to metalworking fluids. Cincinnati, OH: U.S. Department of Health and Human Services, Centers for Disease Control and Prevention, National Institute for Occupational Safety and Health, DHHS (NIOSH) Publication No. 98-102.

NIOSH [2010]. NIOSH pocket guide to chemical hazards. Cincinnati, OH: U.S. Department of Health and Human Services, Centers for Disease Control and Prevention, National Institute for Occupational Safety and Health, DHHS (NIOSH) Publication No. 2010-168c. [http://www.cdc.gov/niosh/npg/]. Date accessed: April 2012.

Rylander R, Jacobs RR [1997]. Endotoxin in the environment. Intl J Occup Environ Health 3(1):S1–S31.

Metalworking Fluid

Air samples for MWFs were collected using 37-mm closed-faced three-piece cassettes containing a tared 2-µm pore-size polytetrafluoroethylene filter and the supporting pad. The sampling train consisted of the 37-mm cassette, a BGI thoracic cyclone, and Tygon® tubing connecting the sampling assembly to SKC Air Check® 2000 air sampling pumps. A sampling rate of 1.6 Lpm was used to collect the thoracic fraction of the aerosol. Each pump was calibrated before and after use. The sampling media was attached to the employee's lapel within the breathing zone (breathing zone is defined as an area in front of the shoulders with a radius of 6 to 9 inches). The samples were analyzed by gravimetric analysis for the thoracic fraction of MWF particulates per NIOSH Method 5524 [NIOSH 2012]. After the filter was gravimetrically weighed, a ternary solvent blend was used to extract the MWF fraction from each sample per NIOSH Method 5524.

Endotoxin

Air samples were collected using an endotoxin-free three-piece 37-mm closed-face cassette, preloaded with 0.45 µm pore-size polycarbonate filters. Samples were collected with AirCheck2000® personal air sampling pumps calibrated at 2 Lpm. Each pump was calibrated before and after use. Endotoxin analysis was performed by a contract laboratory. Samples were analyzed for endotoxin content with the kinetic-chromogenic procedure using the limulus amebocyte lysate assay [Cambrex 2005]. For these analyses, one EU was equivalent to 0.053 nanograms of endotoxin. The limit of detection was 0.025 EU per sample.

Microbial Sampling

Bulk samples of MWFs were collected by filling 1-liter sterile bottles leaving at least 2 inches of headspace. These samples were kept at ambient room temperature and shipped within 2 days to the laboratory for analysis. Each sample was concentrated by a 30-minute centrifuge, and excess fluid was poured off. The concentrate was vortexed for 1 minute and then plated to the appropriate media.

For aerobic bacteria, the media consisted of tryptic soy agar with polysorbate 80 and lecithin and BCYE. Plates were incubated at 23°C ± 2°C for 5 to 7 days and read daily. The media for fungi was yeast malt extract, inhibitory mold agar with gentamicin and chloramphenicol, and BCYE. Plates were incubated at 23°C ± 2°C for 10 days as needed. Plates were read on day 3 to see if it was overgrown, and on days 5 or 7 and day 10.

The media for mycobacteria consisted of BCYE, Middlebrook 7H10, and Mitchison 7H11S. Plates and broth were incubated at 32°C ± 2°C in 7%–10% CO_2 for 4 weeks. Cultures were read at 3 to 5 days and 7 days. If specimens were overgrown, additional dilutions were made. A Ziehl-Neelsen stain of broths was performed at 2–3 weeks and 4 weeks [MSI 2011].

Questionnaire

We recruited employees (exposed) in the aircraft manufacturing building who worked with MWFs and employees in an adjacent building without MWF use (unexposed). Participating employees filled out a questionnaire about demographics, work practices and location, smoking status, and dermal and respiratory symptoms.

The dermatologic questions include questions modified from the Nordic Occupational Skin Questionnaire [Susitaival et al. 2003]. Three questions from the Nordic Occupational Skin Questionnaire were used to determine if participants were atopic (prone to allergic diseases such as asthma, eczema, and allergic rhinitis). A validated question about having an itchy rash that comes and goes for at least six months and has at some time affected skin creases was used to determine a history of atopic dermatitis or eczema [Williams et al. 1994]. A question asking if the participant had ever had hay fever or other symptoms of nasal allergy was used to determine a history of allergic rhinitis. Finally, each participant was asked if he or she had ever had asthma. A participant with a positive answer to any of these three questions was considered atopic.

The respiratory questions include validated questions on asthma symptoms from the European Community Respiratory Health Survey [Grassi et al. 2003]. The questions are: (1) Have you been woken up with a feeling of tightness in your chest at any time in the last 12 months?; (2) Have you had an attack of asthma in the last 12 months?; (3) Are you currently taking any medicine (including inhalers or pumps, aerosols, or tablets) for asthma?; and (4) Have you had wheezing or whistling in your chest at any time in the last 12 months? If participants answered yes to (4) they were asked (a) Have you been at all breathless when the wheezing or whistling noise was present? and (b) Have you had this wheezing or whistling when you did not have a cold? A positive response on any of these questions on the survey has a sensitivity of 75% and a specificity of 80% for asthma symptoms on the basis of a clinical examination with immunoglobulin E testing against common allergens, spirometry, and methacholine challenge testing. We modified these questions by adding the following, "or since beginning your current position if in that position less than 12 months," because some participants had not been in their current position for 12 months. In addition, we added questions about changes in symptoms or medication used on days off work or on vacation. If participants responded that symptoms improved on days off work or on vacation, or that medication use was less frequent on days off or on vacation, then their symptoms were classified as work-related. Finally, if a participant responded positively to any of these questions, he or she was classified as having asthma symptoms.

A question regarding problems with sneezing, runny nose, or blocked nose in the last 12 months probes work-related rhinoconjunctivitis and was adapted from the International Study of Asthma and Allergies in Childhood [Asher et al. 1995]. If participants responded that symptoms improved on days off work or on vacation, then their symptoms were classified as work related. A question regarding more than one episode of illness in the last 12 months with at least two of the following symptoms: cough, wheeze, shortness of breath, or chest tightness was based on diagnostic criteria for HP identified in two prior studies [Fox et al. 1999; Lacasse et al. 2003]. If participants responded positively to this question, they were asked if they had fever or weight loss with these episodes. If they answered yes, they were classified as having symptoms of HP. Participants were also asked if they had pneumonia or chest flu in the last 12 months, and if yes, how many times. This was asked because HP is often misdiagnosed as pneumonia or chest flu. We compared the number of times these illnesses were reported between exposed and unexposed participants.

Workplace information on the questionnaire was used to classify exposure. Participants were defined as exposed to MWFs if they usually worked with MWF in their current job. Other information in the questionnaire included LEV controls, type of MWF supply, PPE use, and hand hygiene questions.

Statistical Analysis

All data were analyzed using SAS 9.2 (SAS Institute Inc., Cary, North Carolina). Data were analyzed by age, sex, smoking status, hours worked per week, work area, and job title. The log binomial regression, Poisson regression, and the Cox proportional hazards model have been recommended to estimate PR [Barros and Hirakata 2003]. The log binomial model directly models the prevalence ratio when the variable is dichotomous [Skov et al. 1998] and was used to estimate PR with 95% CI for dermal and respiratory outcomes in this study. Fitted models for dermal and respiratory outcomes included exposure variables that had greater than 10% change in the PR when included in the model. Chi square or Fisher's exact tests were calculated to determine if there was an association between exposure to MWFs and dermal and respiratory symptoms. The chi square or Fisher's exact tests were used because dichotomous outcomes were compared across 2 groups (exposed and unexposed). The Fisher's exact test was used for sparse data. A P value equal to or less than 0.05 was considered significant. A 95% CI that does not include one was considered significant.

References

Asher MI, Keil U, Anderson HR, Beasley R, Crane J, Martinez F, Mitchell EA, Pearce N, Sibbald B, Stewart AW, Strachan D, Weiland SK, Williams HC [1995]. International Study of Asthma and Allergies in Childhood (ISAAC): rationale and methods. Eur Respir J 8(3):483–491.

Barros AJ, Hirakata VN [2003]. Alternatives for logistic regression in cross-sectional studies: an empirical comparison of models that directly estimate the prevalence ratio. BMC Med Res Methodol 3(1):21.

Cambrex [2005]. Limulus Amebocyte Lysate (LAL), Kinetic-QCL. Catalog Number: 50-650U. Walkersville, MD.

Fox J, Anderson H, Moen T, Gruetzmacher G, Hanrahan L, Fink J [1999]. Metal working fluid-associated hypersensitivity pneumonitis: an outbreak investigation and case-control study. Am J Ind Med 35(1):58–67.

Grassi M, Rezzani C, Biino G, Marinoni A. [2003] Asthma-like symptoms assessment through ECRHS screening questionnaire scoring. J Clin Epidemiol 56(3):238–247.

Lacasse Y, Selman M, Costabel U, Dalphin J, Ando M, Morell F, Erkinjuntti-Pekann R, Muller N, Colby TV, Schuyler M, Cormier Y [2003]. Clinical diagnosis of hypersensitivity pneumonitis. Am J Respir Crit Care Med 168(8):952–958.

MSI [2011]. Microbial analysis – metalworking fluids, Standard operating procedures. Environmental Manual II: SS030.01. Microbiology Specialists, Inc. Houston, TX.

NIOSH [2012]. NIOSH manual of analytical methods (NMAM®), 4th ed. Schlecht PC, O'Connor PF, eds. Cincinnati, OH: U.S. Department of Health and Human Services, Centers for Disease Control and Prevention, National Institute for Occupational Safety and Health, DHHS (NIOSH) Publication 94–113 (August 1994); 1st Supplement Publication 96–135, 2nd Supplement Publication 98–119; 3rd Supplement 2003–154. [http://www.cdc.gov/niosh/docs/2003-154/]. Date accessed: April 2012.

Skov T, Deddens J, Petersen MR, Endahl L [1998]. Prevalence proportion ratios: estimation and hypothesis testing. Int J Epidemiol 27(1):91–95.

Susitaival P, Flyvholm MA, Meding B, Kanerva L, Lindberg M, Svensson A, Olafsson JH [2003]. Nordic Occupational Skin Questionnaire (NOSQ-2002): a new tool for surveying occupational skin diseases and exposure. Contact Dermatitis 49(2):70–76.

Williams HC, Burney PG, Pembroke AC, Hay RJ [1994]. The U.K. Working Party's diagnostic criteria for atopic dermatitis. I. Derivation of a minimum set of discriminators for atopic dermatitis. Br J Dermatol 131(3):383–396.

Appendix C: Tables

Table C1. Production cell machine operators' PBZ air sampling results, engineering control use, and cutting type from May 5–6, 2011

Machine Type	Time (minutes)	Volume (m³)	Thoracic Particulate	Extracted MWF	Enclosure	Mist Collector	Cutting Type
			Concentration (mg/m³)				
Drill	438	0.708	0.11	ND*	None	No	Carbide
Grinder	400	0.650	0.17	ND	Full	Yes	NA†
Grinder	304	0.492	0.16	ND	Partial	Yes	NA
Grinder	407	0.657	0.13	ND	Partial	Yes	NA
Mill	380	0.611	0.29	[0.31]‡	Full	Yes	Carbide
Mill	426	0.680	0.28	ND	None	No	NA
Mill	431	0.696	0.11	ND	Full	No	Carbide
Mill	227	0.367	[0.13]	ND	Partial	No	Carbide
Mill	376	0.607	[0.10]	[0.16]	Partial	No	Carbide
Mill	425	0.699	[0.10]	ND	Full	No	Carbide
Mill drill	365	0.593	[0.06]	ND	None	No	Carbide
Mill drill	399	0.646	0.12	[0.15]	Partial	No	Carbide
Omni mill	370	0.601	0.13	ND	Partial	No	Carbide
Omni mill	385	0.617	[0.11]	ND	None	No	Carbide
Omni mill	401	0.645	[0.09]	ND	Partial	No	Carbide
Omni mill	401	0.653	[0.07]	ND	Partial	No	Carbide
Omni mill	319	0.519	[0.05]	ND	Partial	No	Carbide
Turning	367	0.595	0.20	ND	Partial	Yes	Carbide
Turning	379	0.613	0.14	ND	Partial§	Yes, but off	Carbide
Turning	421	0.689	0.14	ND	Full	Yes	Ceramic
Turning	398	0.637	[0.09]	ND	Full	Yes	Carbide
Turning	400	0.639	[0.09]	ND	Partial	Yes	Carbide
Turning	381	0.621	[0.08]	ND	Full	Yes	Carbide
Turning	361	0.584	[0.07]	[0.19]	Partial	Yes, but off	Both¶
Turning	444	0.688	[0.06]	ND	Partial	Yes	Both
Turning	441	0.712	[0.05]	ND	Partial	No	Carbide
Turning	419	0.676	[0.04]	ND	Partial	Yes	Both
VTL	379	0.615	0.21	ND	Full	Yes	Both
VTL	426	0.687	0.14	ND	Partial	Yes	Both
VTL	390	0.626	0.14	ND	Partial	Yes	Ceramic
VTL	392	0.635	0.12	ND	None	No	Carbide
VTL	411	0.668	0.12	ND	Full	Unknown	Ceramic
VTL	434	0.696	0.11	ND	Full	Yes	Both
VTL	333	0.538	[0.11]	ND	Full	Yes	Both
VTL	415	0.649	[0.11]	ND	None	No	Carbide
VTL	416	0.675	[0.10]	ND	Partial	Yes	Carbide
VTL	421	0.683	[0.09]	ND	Partial	Yes	Carbide
VTL	412	0.661	[0.09]	ND	Partial	Yes	Both

Table C1. Production cell machine operators' PBZ air sampling results, engineering control use, and cutting type from May 5–6, 2011 (continued)

Machine Type	Time (minutes)	Volume (m³)	Thoracic Particulate	Extracted MWF	Enclosure	Mist Collector	Cutting Type
			Concentration (mg/m³)				
VTL	237	0.385	[0.07]	ND	Partial	Yes, but off	Carbide
VTL	247	0.399	[0.07]	ND	Partial	Yes	Carbide
VTL	427	0.685	[0.07]	ND	Partial	Yes	Carbide
VTL	411	0.666	[0.07]	ND	Partial	No	Carbide
VTL	427	0.695	[0.04]	ND	None	No	Carbide
Hot oil flush	437	0.705	0.12	ND	NA	NA	NA
Hot oil flush	298	0.484	[0.08]	ND	NA	NA	NA
Stand-alone machine	388	0.620	0.13	ND	None	Yes	NA
NIOSH REL (10-hour TWA)			0.4	None			
OSHA PEL			None	None			
ACGIH TLV			None	None			
MDC** (mg/m³)			0.03	0.14			
MQC** (mg/m³)			0.12	0.50			

*ND – not detected
†NA – not applicable
‡Concentrations between the MDC and MQC are shown in brackets to acknowledge that there is more uncertainty associated with these values than with concentrations above the MQC.
§Observed that enclosure was left open when machine was operating
¶Both carbide and ceramic cutting
**Based on an average air volume of 0.625 m³

Table C2. Area air sampling results for MWFs on May 5–6, 2011

	Day 1				Day 2			
	Time	Volume	Concentration (mg/m^3)		Time	Volume	Concentration (mg/m^3)	
			Thoracic	Extracted			Thoracic	Extracted
Location	(minutes)	(m^3)	Particulate	MWF	(minutes)	(m^3)	Particulate	MWF
Large parts	468	0.755	0.17	[0.17]*	417	0.676	0.12	ND†
North central system	432	0.692	0.13	ND	416	0.661	0.13	ND
Milling	376	0.607	0.13	ND	430	0.695	0.24	[0.22]
Mill drill	NA‡	NA	NA	NA	348	0.565	0.16	ND
Building 800	271	NA§	NA§	NA§	346	0.564	[0.07]	ND
MDC¶ (mg/m^3)			0.03	0.14			0.03	0.14
MQC¶ (mg/m^3)			0.12	0.50			0.12	0.50

*Concentrations between the MDC and MQC are shown in brackets to acknowledge that there is more uncertainty associated with these values than with concentrations above the MQC.
†ND – not detected
‡NA – not applicable
§Missing information
¶Based on an average air volume of 0.625 m^3

Table C3. Area endotoxin air sampling results on May 5–6, 2011

Location	Time (minutes)	Volume (m^3)	Concentration (EU/m^3)
Mill	376	0.745	2.7
VTL	382	0.76	2.6
Hot oil flush	198	0.40	1.9
North Central System	431	0.86	1.7
VTL	375	0.74	1.5
Omni mill	385	0.76	1.6
VTL	194	0.39	1.4
Turning machine	371	0.74	1.3
Mill	320	0.63	0.85
Turning machine	318	0.63	0.83
VTL	315	0.63	0.69
Turning machine	304	0.47	0.61
VTL	375	0.74	0.55
VTL	298	0.59	0.48
VTL	318	0.63	0.46
Drill mill	364	0.73	0.45
Grinder	319	0.64	0.42
Mean			1.18
Meeting room sample 1	176	0.53	0.23
Meeting room sample 2	244	0.80	0.24

Appendix D: Tips on preventing dermatitis

Avoiding irritants and allergens, in addition to wet work, is the first step in dermatitis prevention. Liberal use of skin moisturizers helps to prevent contact dermatitis by maintaining a healthy skin barrier and also helps to repair this barrier if it has been compromised [Chew and Maibach 2003]. The following list provides strategies in the prevention of occupational contact dermatitis:

- Identifying irritants and allergens
- Substituting chemicals that are less irritating or allergenic
- Establishing engineering controls to reduce exposure
- Emphasizing personal and occupational hygiene
- Establishing educational programs to increase awareness in the workplace
- Utilizing PPE, such as gloves and special clothing [NIOSH 1988]

Chemical changes in industrial materials have been beneficial. For example, the addition of ferrous sulfate to cement to reduce the hexavalent chromium content has been effective in reducing occupational allergic contact dermatitis in Europe.

Protective gloves can reduce or eliminate skin exposure to hazardous substances if used correctly, but may actually cause or worsen hand dermatitis (by permeation and penetration) if selected poorly and used improperly (by contamination) [Foo et al. 2006]. Gloves may occlude irritants or allergens next to the skin, and PPE components may directly irritate the skin, so the correct use of PPE is at least as important as the correct selection of materials [Kwon et al. 2006].

Similarly, the excessive pursuit of personal hygiene in the workplace may actually lead to misuse of soaps and detergents and cause irritant contact dermatitis. Proper hand washing methods and adequate moisturizing are valuable in preventing contact dermatitis [Warshaw et al. 2003]. The effectiveness of barrier creams is controversial because data on the protective nature of these topical products during actual working conditions involving high-risk exposures are limited.

Educating the workforce about skin care, exposures, and PPE use is an especially important measure in the prevention of occupational contact dermatitis [Schwanitz et al. 2003; Loffler et al. 2006; Weisshaar et al. 2006].

The following list provides tips on proper hand washing [Warshaw et al. 2003]:

- Avoid hot water; use lukewarm or cool water instead.
- Use mild cleansers without perfume, coloring, or antibacterial agents.
- Pat hands dry, especially between fingers.
- Apply skin moisturizer generously after hand washing and repeat throughout the day.
- Avoid rubbing, scrubbing, the use of washcloths, and the overuse of soap and water.

The following list provides tips for the workplace [Warshaw et al. 2003]:

- Remove rings before work.

- Wear protective gloves in cold weather and for dusty work.

- Wear tight-fitting leather gloves for frictional exposures.

- When performing "wet work," wear cotton gloves under vinyl or other nonlatex gloves.

- Avoid immersing hands; use running water if possible.

References

Chew AI, Maibach HI [2003]. Occupational issues of irritant contact dermatitis. Int Arch Occup Environ Health 76(5):339–346.

Foo CC, Goon AT, Leow YH, Goh CL [2006]. Adverse skin reactions to personal protective equipment against severe acute respiratory sundrome-a descriptive study in Singapore. Contact Dermatitis 55(5):291–294.

Kwon S, Campbell LS, Zirwas MJ [2006]. Role of protective gloves in the causation and treatment of occupational irritant contact dermatitis. J Am Acad Dermatol 55(5):891–896.

Loffler H, Bruckner T, Diepgen T, Effendy I [2006]. Primary prevention in health care employees: a prospective intervention study with a 3-year training period. Contact Dermatitis 54(4):202–209.

NIOSH [1988]. Proposed national strategy for the prevention of leading work-related diseases and injuries: Dermatological conditions. Cincinnati, OH: U.S. Department of Health and Human Services, Centers for Disease Control and Prevention, National Institute for Occupational Safety and Health, DHHS (NIOSH), Publication No. 89-136.

Schwanitz HJ, Riel U, Schlesinger T, Bock M, Skudlik C, Wulfhorst B [2003]. Skin care management: educational aspects. Int Arch Occup Environ Health 76(5):374–381.

Warshaw E, Lee G, Storrs FJ [2003]. Hand dermatitis: a review of clinical features, therapeutic options and long-term outcomes. Am J Contact Dermat 14(3):119–137.

Weisshaer E, Radulescu M, Bock M, Albrecht U, Diepgen TL [2006]. Educational and dermatological aspects of secondary individual prevention in healthcare workers. Contact Dermatitis 54(5):254–260.

This page left intentionally blank.

This page left intentionally blank.

ACKNOWLEDGMENTS AND AVAILABILITY OF REPORT

The Hazard Evaluations and Technical Assistance Branch (HETAB) of the National Institute for Occupational Safety and Health (NIOSH) conducts field investigations of possible health hazards in the workplace. These investigations are conducted under the authority of Section 20(a)(6) of the Occupational Safety and Health Act of 1970, 29 U.S.C. 669(a)(6) which authorizes the Secretary of Health and Human Services, following a written request from any employer or authorized representative of employees, to determine whether any substance normally found in the place of employment has potentially toxic effects in such concentrations as used or found. HETAB also provides, upon request, technical and consultative assistance to federal, state, and local agencies; labor; industry; and other groups or individuals to control occupational health hazards and to prevent related trauma and disease.

Mention of any company or product does not constitute endorsement by NIOSH. In addition, citations to websites external to NIOSH do not constitute NIOSH endorsement of the sponsoring organizations or their programs or products. Furthermore, NIOSH is not responsible for the content of these websites. All Web addresses referenced in this document were accessible as of the publication date.

This report was prepared by Lilia Chen and Francisco Meza of HETAB, and Naomi Hudson of Surveillance Branch, Division of Surveillance, Hazard Evaluations and Field Studies. Industrial hygiene field assistance was provided by Diana Ceballos, James Couch, Matthew Dahm, and Todd Niemeier. Industrial hygiene equipment and logistical support were provided by Donald Booher and Karl Feldmann. Medical field assistance was provided by Carlos Aristeguieta, Marie De Perio, Chad Dowell, Judith Eisenberg, Stefanie Evans, Kemka Hekerem, Melody Kawamoto, Charles Mueller, Elena Page, Robert McCleery, Alysha Meyers, Jessica Ramsey, Loren Tapp, Allison Tepper, and Douglas Wiegand. Statistical analysis was provided by Naomi Hudson. Analytical support was provided by Bureau Veritas North America (Novi, Michigan), Microbiology Specialists Incorporated (Houston, Texas), and EMLab P&K (Cherry Hill, New Jersey). Health communication assistance was provided by Stefanie Evans. Editorial assistance was provided by Ellen Galloway. Desktop publishing was performed by Greg Hartle and Mary Winfree.

Copies of this report have been sent to employee and management representatives, the state health department, and the Occupational Safety and Health Administration Regional Office. This report is not copyrighted and may be freely reproduced. The report may be viewed and printed at http://www.cdc.gov/niosh/hhe/. Copies may be purchased from the National Technical Information Service at 5825 Port Royal Road, Springfield, Virginia 22161.

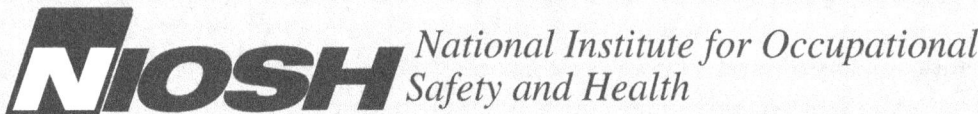 National Institute for Occupational Safety and Health

Delivering on the Nation's promise: Safety and health at work for all people through research and prevention.

To receive NIOSH documents or information about occupational safety and health topics, contact NIOSH at:

1-800-CDC-INFO (1-800-232-4636)

TTY: 1-888-232-6348

E-mail: cdcinfo@cdc.gov

or visit the NIOSH web site at: **www.cdc.gov/niosh.**

For a monthly update on news at NIOSH, subscribe to NIOSH eNews by visiting **www.cdc.gov/niosh/eNews.**

SAFER · HEALTHIER · PEOPLE™

www.ingramcontent.com/pod-product-compliance
Lightning Source LLC
Chambersburg PA
CBHW080917290526
45795CB00007BA/2556